HOW DO YO
LET US COUNT THE WAYS.

- How often and how loudly do you snore? (Only your bed partner knows for sure.)
- Can your snoring be heard in other rooms? In other counties?
- Does your snoring stop at times while you sleep? Does it ever sound to your partner as if you've stopped breathing?
- Has snoring ever caused you to wake up suddenly?
- Are you often sleepy during the day?

SCORE YOUR SNORE
TO KNOW YOUR CURE.

Stop the Snoring!

RALPH SCHOENSTEIN

CONSULTING EDITOR
YOSEF P. KRESPI, M.D.

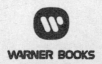

WARNER BOOKS

A Time Warner Company

WARNER BOOKS EDITION

Cover design by Irving Freeman
Cover photograph by Telegraph/FPG International

Warner Books, Inc.
1271 Avenue of the Americas
New York, NY 10020

Visit our Web site at
http://warnerbooks.com

W A Time Warner Company

Printed in the United States of America

First Printing: November, 1997

10 9 8 7 6 5 4 3 2 1

The author thanks these eminent physicians who graciously contributed their time and knowledge to this book:

Neil B. Kavey, M.D., F.A.C.S.
Director of Sleep Disorders
Columbia-Presbyterian Medical Center
New York City

Gabriele M. Barthlen, M.D., F.A.C.S.
Former Director of Sleep Medicine
Mount Sinai Hospital
New York City

David O. Goldfarb, M.D., F.A.C.S.
Chief of Otolaryngology
The Medical Center at Princeton
Princeton, New Jersey

Dennis R. Bailey, D.D.S., F.A.G.D.
Diplomate, American Board of Orofacial Pain
Hamilton, New Jersey

Steven D. Handler, M.D.
Otolaryngology
The Children's Hospital
Philadelphia

Arlene H. Markowitz, M.D., F.A.C.S.
Otolaryngology
New York City

And

Susan Devereux

PREFACE

You are about to read a book that will put you to sleep—the right way, that is.

Sleep disorders affect millions of people, and the major sleep disorder is snoring. That, of course, is why you bought this book: to save your marriage or your sanity or both. Well, I'm happy to say that you and your spouse are on your way to quiet sleep because this book presents the last word on snoring.

The last word on snoring is *cure*. And in these pages, you'll find the right cure for the particular kind of snoring that you or your spouse does. Yes, there are different kinds of snoring and they call for different treatments. Even small children snore, but we're not concerned with them in this book. They merely need to have their tonsils removed, but it's not that simple for their fathers.

For too many years, from Mark Twain to the Three Stooges, snoring has been an easy joke; but the joke isn't funny to all the victims of snoring and *their* victims, their mates. In my work in treating sleep disorders, I have seen the despair of deeply afflicted snorers as they move from one so-called cure to another, none of which works.

In this book, however, are the latest cures that *do* work: precisely how they work and what are their costs and any possible drawbacks. Moreover, as entertaining counterpoint for all the medical expertise, Ralph Schoenstein gives his personal odyssey of seeking a cure for his own snoring; and with that odyssey, he weaves tales of other snorers he has known.

All of these tales move the book toward the revelation you have desperately sought for so long: how to bring peace to your pillow and the one beside you.

Thoroughly up to date, this book reflects the constantly developing science of otolaryngology. For example, just before the book went to press, a new homeopathic pill that supposedly cures snoring was put on the market. I could not, however, even *think* of recommending such a pill, because it hasn't been properly tested in standard clinical trials. And that's the key: this book recommends *only* the treatments that have been thoroughly tested and it tells you why the others won't work.

And so, stay awake now for some good reading. You're about to learn the answer you've been seeking and also have a great deal of pleasure along the way.

                                Yosef P. Krespi, M.D., F.A.C.S.

CONTENTS

The minute my husband hits the pillow, it's as if someone had started a power motor inches from my head. I poke. I plead. I say, "Why me?"

—Sleepless in St. Louis

CHAPTER ONE

Can This Marriage Be Saved?

Every night in America, forty million women have to make a decision about moving that has nothing to do with packing china. For each of these women, the equally poignant choices are: Should *she* leave the bedroom where her husband is snoring or preparing to snore? Or should she evict *him* to avoid another long night of black sound? As my own wife, Judy, has tenderly said, "Either you stop breathing or one of us has to get out."

Snoring is a greater threat to marriage than an obnoxious teenager. It has led to divorce and gunfire, not always in that order. A Texan named John Wesley Hardin once fired a shot through a wall at a snorer in the next room and killed him, teaching him a lesson considered by such women as Tauba Heidenreich, the wife of a singer-snorer, who said, "I wouldn't mind taking a pillow and putting it over his face, if I thought I could get away with it. Instead, I hit the couch and start thinking of ways to torture him."

"Snoring is the biggest problem for marriages that we

see," says Dr. Rosalind Cartwright, director of Sleep Disorder Services at Chicago's St. Luke's Medical Center. "The man's wife has left the bed because of his snoring and he wants her back."

In more alarming words, Dr. Neil B. Kavey, director of the Sleep Disorders Center at New York's Columbia Presbyterian Medical Center, says, "Doctors used to say, 'If you have a good marriage, it will survive snoring.' But this is simply not true."

And the marriage is never saved merely by poking your dysfunctional darling in the dead of night. Instead, you might be driven to consider calling a lawyer in the morning. In 1971, snoring was declared legal grounds for divorce. A woman no longer was obliged to stay tied to someone she had to keep rotating as if running an all-night barbecue.

The silencing of a snorer—without pistol or chloroform, that is—has long been a miracle as eagerly sought as the Fountain of Youth. In fact, Ponce de Leon's wife said to him, "Try making yourself about three—or *any* age that's presnoring." For centuries, there have been desperate attempts to save snore-filled marriages with cannonballs, bricks, straitjackets, harnesses, neck-extenders, face masks, face-molders, nose clips, herbs, and mystical rites. Did a sleepless Inca wife finally just decide to toss the guy into a volcano?

My own wife keeps shaking me, even though she poignantly knows that a man who snores on his stomach has nowhere to go. Now, however, if she stays with me long enough to read this book, she will have her first chance to sleep for more than twenty.

Because of what is between these covers, a wife at last will be able to put *herself* between covers beside the noiseless mouth of her dreams.

My wife hasn't had a decent night's sleep in twenty years. If I stop snoring, she frantically pokes me to see if I'm still alive.
—MONITORED IN DUBUQUE

CHAPTER TWO

A Little Too Much Night Music

W hat is snoring?

This is hardly a question from a PhD exam, but we still should start by answering it—from *Webster's New International Dictionary,* which can be used to raise the head of a snorer's bed in an old-fashioned treatment that this book will go far beyond. *Webster's* says that to snore is *To breathe during sleep with a rough, hoarse noise, due to vibration of the uvula and soft palate.*

And you thought that the uvula was a river in Latvia instead of the V-shaped bag that hangs from the back of your soft palate, which is the tissue extending from both sides of the uvula that separates the back of the throat from the back of the nose. The longer your uvula is, the smaller is your upper airway and the more likely you are to have the flutter that is snoring.

All snoring is caused by some degree of blockage in the upper airway.

To make sure that *Webster's* wasn't guessing, I went to *The Columbia Encyclopedia*, which says that snoring is

> *Rough, vibratory sounds accompanying breathing during sleep. The noisy breathing is associated with the relaxation of the palate and an open mouth. Any obstruction interfering with normal breathing through the nose may produce such sounds during sleep. In some individuals, snoring is avoided by sleeping on the side.*

But in many others, it is *not*.

That, as I've said, is how my wife, Judy, sleeps: on the side. The rest of the time, she's awake, thinking of the uvulas she could have married and counting decibels instead of sheep. A first-rate snorer can hit eighty decibels, just ten below a ringing phone.

When *I* sleep on my side, I snore on my side, as Judy has pointed out between yawns at breakfast.

"You hit the Richter scale last night," she said a few days ago. "You've really got to do something about that fault line in your nose."

"Honey, I feel *terrible* about it," I said. "Of course, I've never heard it. You know, Mark Twain wrote about snoring and he wondered why a snorer can never hear himself."

"In his current condition, Mark Twain could've heard *you*. It sounds as though someone is mowing the bed."

"Did you know that *twenty* Presidents snored?"

"I wouldn't have voted for any of them."

"Snoring isn't the *nose,* by the way: it's *mouth* breathing when your throat relaxes in sleep and your tongue falls back to the airway and causes vibration in the soft tissue just above the pharynx. See how much I've already learned?"

"You don't have to go on *Jeopardy*; just find a way to stop it."

"I *will*. My great quest has begun!"

"Maybe I'll make a tape of your snoring to help you. Susan is taping Al. Betsy can't tape Mike because he just moved out."

"I wonder what's proper etiquette today. Should the man or the woman move out?"

Judy smiled through a yawn. "I'll have to ask my support group. Mention snoring to them—or to *anyone*—and the responses are electric."

"Yes, so many people snore. Remember that movie, *Heavenly Body*? William Powell falls asleep on Hedy Lamarr's shoulder and starts to snore. Winston *Churchill* snored. Washington and Roosevelt, too. Even *Lincoln* snored. But new treatments have come out and one of them *has* to work for me."

"I don't want you having surgery."

"I think there are things that don't call for bleeding."

"You know what Sam has to do for Laurie? He usually goes to sleep in another room because he's afraid his snoring will wake her. But sometimes, in the middle of the night, he gambles and comes back 'cause he loves being beside her. But he's really just replacing her—it's a domino effect— because then she's out of there after attacking him for a while with her elbow and her foot. Just *imagine:* most of the *country* is on the move every night."

"It's something you never read about in *Travel and Leisure*."

My wife has a lovely little nose and still she snores. That she is a woman has nothing to do with her ability to fill the night with sound.

—ROLE REVERSED IN SANTA FE

CHAPTER THREE

All the Causes of the Noise

Before we plunge into my medical and personal exploration of all the treatments for snoring, before we explore both clinical genius and over-the-counter junk, let us speak more about the cause and the victims—the victims, that is, who transmit, not those who receive.

What is the most common cause of snoring?

A man who falls asleep, you say.

Yes, of course, even though about 10 percent of snorers are women, a figure that rises after menopause. Premenopausal women are protected from snoring by the hormone progesterone, a respiratory stimulant that seems to stabilize the muscles of the upper airway. And so, before menopause, female snorers are outnumbered by males about thirty to one. In shattering the peace of the night, there will never be sexual equality: men have thicker tissue in their throats. Snoring and raising toilet seats are the only things in the world that men will always do better than women.

A study of female patients in one Canadian clinic revealed that 86 percent of them said their husbands snored. About 25 percent of all men snore every night and 45 percent of all men over fifty snore to some degree. Moreover, there is a progressive increase: in the age group between forty-one and sixty-four, 60 percent of men snore almost every night. In decibel count, an older man often snores his age.

Normal speech is about forty decibels of loudness and a baby crying about sixty. Loud snorers, however, can hit eighty decibels, which is about the same volume as a jackhammer or the barking of a dog.

"We call it heroic snoring," one doctor told me.

What every wife wants, of course, is a quiet coward.

In the field of throaty heroics, the Medal of Honor is held by an Englishman named Melvin Switzer, who snored at ninety-one decibels in 1992 and set the world's record—perhaps. Because snoring is not an Olympic event, Switzer's title is open to challenge; other measurements have shown that some snorers produce noise as loud as a jet taking off. Every night, millions of wives are sleeping on a runway, but the flight never leaves.

In adults, there are two basic causes of snoring: relaxed muscles in the throat and masses partially blocking it. In sleep, particularly in deep sleep, the throat muscles relax and the tongue falls back, causing vibration and a sound that is funny only in Laurel and Hardy films. Because gravity moves the tongue in the wrong direction, most snoring occurs when the sleeper is on his back.

I, however, have never been able to sleep on my back or even my side, which has always struck me as a transitional position. I sleep on my stomach, but still manage to avoid the sounds of silence and test Judy's love for me. Snoring, in fact, may be the ultimate test of love. The marriage vow should be revised, even though "till death or snoring do you part" has a less poetic ring.

Estimates about the percentage of snorers in the population cannot, of course, be precise, but doctors feel that about 45 percent of all adults snore from time to time, always because their tongues make a kind of kazoo against the floppy tissues at the backs of their throats. The farther back the tongue drops, the more vibrating, or snoring, occurs. Our tongues can get us into trouble when we're asleep as well as awake.

The size of your uvula is a fundamental factor in whether or not you'll be driving your loved one loony at night, for central to snoring is the uvula's fluttering. *You* remember the uvula: that fleshy lobe dangling from the back of the throat. The average one is about a quarter-inch, but some people have uvulas four times that size and Richard Simmons has no workout to make them smaller.

Another big factor in snoring is obesity. Overweight people are three times more likely to snore than people of average weight because their bulkiness extends throughout their bodies. *This* is where a workout can help: if you do aerobics during the day, you just might get more air at night.

Thin people do snore too, of course. *I* snore every night and yet I look like something that might be hanging in a medical school.

Because smoking is deadly for the lungs, the Surgeon General doesn't bother to mention that smoking also swells the mucous membranes in the throat and therefore narrows the upper airway. Other upper-airway blockers are large tonsils and large adenoids, as well as anything obstructing the nose that makes you breathe through your mouth at night: congestion from a cold, hay fever, polyps, or a deviated septum, which is the tissue separating the two sides of the nasal cavity. Nasal breathing *can* cause snoring, but it's a greater achievement to snore that way.

Moreover, alcohol, sleeping pills, antihistamines, and aging also reduce the tone of the muscles in the throat; and so, you can reduce the potential for snoring by not drinking, taking bedtime pills, or getting older. You can also start exercising, for sedentary people are more likely to snore than those who are physically fit.

To sum it up, some combination of the following conditions can make you sound like a car missing a muffler: your weight, your general physical condition, your sleeping position, the drift of your tongue during sleep, the size and floppiness of your uvula and soft palate, the size of your upper airway, the size of your jaw, the size of your tonsils and adenoids, your nasal congestion, your nasal design, your bedtime medications, your intake of alcohol, and even your genes. My father, the child of Hungarians, snored; and my mother's father, the child of Czechs, snored too. What Judy hears are sounds that have come through Ellis Island.

Snoring did not start in middle Europe, of course. Adam may have snored in the Garden of Eden, particularly if there was pollen in the air and if he slept on his back; but the word "snore" does happen to be derived from the low German *snorren* and the medieval Dutch *snarren,* words that mean "to drone" and "to hum."

If you had to describe the average humming drone, he would be an overweight man of fifty with too much tissue all over the place.

"Whenever I see a lot of extra tissue in the throat, I say, 'I'll bet you snore,' " says Dr. Bill Moran, spokesman for the American Academy of Otolaryngology.

Well, get ready to clear your throat, for here comes all the help that I have found for you. As the jazzmen like to say: Let's turn on the quiet.

My wife and I haven't slept in the same bed for years. The trouble was, she could still hear me.

—AWESOME IN PHOENIX

CHAPTER FOUR

It Can Damage More Than Your Marriage

As I began my layman's exploration of snoring, feeling like the Marco Polo of the soft palate, I learned that there are different degrees of it and that treatment should be tailored to the individual after an office exam by a doctor or an overnight study at a sleep disorders center to reveal the precise disruption in the intake of air. You may have thought that a sleep disorders center is a motel full of rappers, but there is a kind where people are wired in another way and we will visit it later in the book.

In degree, snoring ranges from "social snoring," which is snoring acceptable at dinner parties, all the way up through heroic snoring to a condition called obstructive sleep apnea, when the airway is totally blocked and breathing stops for ten seconds or more. The danger of sleep apnea is losing not your wife but your life: having to wake up several times a night to search for your breath raises your blood pressure, decreases the oxygen in your blood, and strains your heart and lungs.

"Doctors should *never* trivialize snoring by telling a patient, 'Oh, I snore, too,' " says Dr. Neil B. Kavey at New York's Columbia Presbyterian Medical Center. "Instead, they should find out exactly what *kind* of snoring is being done. Is it merely disruptive to the partner or dangerous to the individual?"

And so, you must first determine your snorer's grade—and whether there's a chance that he is taking life pass-fail.

The most benign snoring is the soft variety that disturbs no one and can even have a certain guttural charm. Judy sometimes snores this way, a gentle buzz I find lovable, as if a bee has gotten stuck in our sheets.

A less endearing buzz, however, is the one she hears from me: a loud and generally even kind that affects not my health but her sleep, a kind that has moved her to try earplugs. Even with the plugs, however, she still was able to hear my snoring, though the volume had dropped; but she stopped using them because she feared that she wouldn't hear the smoke alarm or a comet hitting the living room.

My study of snoring has made me both learned and lunatic. Whenever Judy tells me at breakfast that I was snoring last night, I reply, "Was it all *regular?*"

"Yes," she says. "My regular way to go nuts."

"*You* know what I mean: Was it all smooth and even?"

"You mean did you die? No, you didn't die."

"That's good to hear. Dr. Kavey told me that even normal snorers—"

Which isn't *you.*

"—can stop breathing as often as twenty times an hour. Are you *sure* I didn't stop breathing every once in a while?"

"No, but if you keep this up, I might try to arrange it. For the nine hundredth time, your snoring *isn't* appian."

"I hope it's not apnea either."

The next most severe degree of snoring is the heroic with

syncopation, a form called hypopnea, which sounds like a spring blossom but is really a loud, irregular snore that advertises a brief blockage. In hypopnea, a word from the Greek meaning "less breathing," there is decreased air flow through the nose and mouth of at least ten seconds: the snorer keeps making efforts to draw air through his partially blocked airway. It is not a pretty sight for any pillow, particularly one in your bed.

Even less attractive is the worst snoring of all, apnea, the Greek word that means "no breathing." Because the lungs are suddenly getting no air, the brain tells the body to wake up just enough to tighten the muscles and unblock the airway, a jump start that can happen many times a night. Both apnea and hypopnea cause a loud snort, a brief awakening that restores muscle tone, raises the oxygen level again, and scares small children passing by.

The lack of sleep and fresh air from apnea can strain both the heart and lungs, causing premature heart disease, high blood pressure, and stroke. When an extremely overweight young man like John Candy dies in his sleep, apnea may have been the cause.

Moreover, apnea also can weaken the immune system and cause depression; and, because it deprives you of sleep, it can make you take a little nap while driving, for daytime sleepiness is another of its effects. There is a great consciousness today about drunk driving, but considerably less consciousness about *unconscious* driving caused by an oxygen-lowered night.

"If untreated, apnea can kill 35 percent of patients within five years," says Dr. Raymond C. Rosen, director of the Sleep Disorders Center of Robert Wood Johnson Hospital in New Brunswick, New Jersey.

Every year, between two and three thousand Americans die in their sleep from cardiac arrest caused by sleep apnea.

One way or another, sleep apnea kills thirty-eight thousand Americans every year, not enough for a telethon but enough to make every snorer want to learn if his buzz is just a nuisance or perhaps a death sentence. There is also a rare condition called central sleep apnea, a failure of the brain's automatic breathing center that makes sleep permanent; but more than 90 percent of apneas are caused by obstruction in the upper airway, obstruction that can sometimes stop breathing for more than a minute.

The long breathing stoppages from apnea do not always happen, but the short ones do and they come in alarming multiples.

"It's like having a cork stuck in your throat two or three hundred times a night," one snorer says.

Of the twenty million Americans who have obstructive sleep apnea, the typical sufferer is an overweight man who sleeps on his back, has a small jaw, and a small opening at the back of his throat. If you are such a man, do not run out to update your will. Instead, run out to your doctor and be ready to get an A on the following quiz:

CHAPTER FIVE

Get Your Degree!
A Snoring Test

And here's the test for your degree—your degree of snoring, that is. You *must* learn it before you can find the precise treatment that's right for you.

Only your doctor can report the meaning of your score. Your marriage, your health, perhaps even your *life,* may depend on your knowing it.

- How often and how loudly do you snore? You'll have to get the answer from your bed partner, if you still have one. Bring her to the doctor's evaluation.
- Can your snoring be heard from other rooms? From other counties?
- Does the snoring stop at times while you sleep? Does it ever sound to your partner as though you've stopped breathing?
- Do you gasp in your sleep?
- Has snoring ever caused you to wake up suddenly?
- What is your usual sleep position? If it's sleeping on

your back, do you snore only in that position? If you change your position, does the snoring get better or worse or stay the same?

- Do you drink alcohol in the evening?
- Do you smoke?
- Do you take antihistamines, sleeping pills, or sedatives? If so, how often?
- How many hours a night do you usually sleep?
- When you awaken, do you feel refreshed?
- When driving, do you feel waves of sleepiness that enable you to play roadway roulette?
- Are you often sleepy at other times during the day?

CHAPTER SIX

If You Need a Bigger Exam

By having your doctor score your test and then examine you in the office, you will learn the specific nature of your snoring: whether it is apnea, hypopnea, or nonthreateningly heroic, whether it is dangerous or simply a harmless way to unhinge the mind of a loved one. If, however, the doctor's exam isn't probing enough to be certain about the seriousness of your snoring, then you may have to spend a night at a sleep disorders center to learn if you have apnea. These centers are all over the country, as you'll see in the back of the book.

What is the routine at such a pajama party?

After a preliminary exam by an otolaryngologist at the center, you report there with your overnight bag, which should contain your toothbrush, pajamas or nightgown, pillow, books, stuffed animals—whatever will help you sleep comfortably. The center will want you to follow your normal bedtime routine, except for using alcohol or medication. You will probably be given a private room, though certain centers may give you a roommate. Will his snoring keep you from getting to sleep to learn how *you* snore? Try counting the bill—about $2,000. A night at the Hyatt is cheaper, but insurance won't pay for it. Insurance, however, will probably pay all or most of your sleep center expense because the company knows that finding out if you have apnea is more than getting a nose job.

If you're a snorer but still not concerned about having apnea, consider these sobering thoughts: About 80 percent of the people with apnea are *unaware* they have a condition that can drain their energy, cheerfulness, wakefulness, and concentration during the day and, at *any* time, their lives. One study of sixty-four people in Virginia revealed that those with sleep apnea had seven times more automobile accidents than the average driver; and one-quarter of them said that they fell asleep at the wheel at least once a week.

And you're afraid of *flying*.

Because apnea tends to run in families, a pattern of it in your own family should move you to have an examination at a sleep disorders center, especially if you're a man and also getting older. Apnea, like all other snoring, worsens with age. And which of us is going in the other direction?

When you go to sleep at the center, sensors with wires leading to a polysomnograph are attached to your forehead, nose, chin, and chest so the machine can record the activity of your heart, lungs, and brain, the movements of your muscles, the air flow from your nose and mouth, and the level of oxygen in your blood. Your body's movements will also be videotaped and your snoring recorded.

If the polysomnograph detects a lower level of oxygen in your blood during the night, then the following day you are liable to lose focus, judgment, and reaction time. Your judgment is particularly bad in thinking that you slept all night. The day after a night of severe snoring, you are sleepy because innumerable times the buildup of unexhaled carbon dioxide became an alarm that tightened your muscles and brought you either fully awake or into a light, restless sleep. In other words, your night's sleep was a few hundred naps.

Sleep center directors say that most people have no trouble falling asleep at the center, but there is room for doubt. Falling asleep with wires attached to you and a camera running is a routine that's easier for someone in the space program. However, when you finally do get to sleep, a technician will be watching monitors throughout the night to make sure the equipment is working and that your breathing is working, too. If you happen to have any dangerous spell of apnea during the night, he will open your airway with a device that we'll soon examine.

"Sleep study isn't to learn about the *noise* of snoring," says Dr. Neil B. Kavey. "For that, we pretty much have to take the partner's word; in fact, the snorer may not make too many sounds on the night we study him. The point of sleep study is to define the exact disruption of air flow. Even in apnea, there's a whole spectrum: there's a big difference between 60 apneas with oxygen levels of 88 percent and 200 apneas with oxygen levels of 58 percent. Either way, of course, apnea nips away at a person's cardiac function through the years, and also strains the vessels in the brain. Without enough oxygen, you're like an engine knocking from low octane. The apnea sufferer is usually an overweight person, but it doesn't *have* to be. We watch for small jaws, thick tongues, and overbites."

How dismayed I was by those words! I have always been enchanted by women with slight overbites, no matter what the size of their tongues. Confirming my dental desire, Judy has said that every man likes a woman with a slight overbite. And now to hear Dr. Kavey say that the vision of my youthful dreams, Gene Tierney, might have shattered those dreams with snores if her sensuously protruding teeth and small but bewitching jaw had been on a pillow beside me.

If your doctor finds no apnea after your night at the sleep center, he may say that you need only certain changes in your lifestyle to reduce your snoring, changes such as getting exercise, losing weight, and doing less drinking. If you *don't* feel inclined to make such changes, then all you can do to save your marriage is give your wife earplugs, or make sure that she always goes to sleep first, or find her a nice room down the hall.

However, if you want to do more than just *reduce* your snoring, you can use one of the techniques or devices in the chapters to come. This book is to let you *cure* snoring, not just mask it or lessen it or flee from it, so we'll now move on to the cures that are available to you.

The first one just happens to *be* a mask, but nothing you ever wore for Halloween.

First I poke him with my toe. Then I poke him with my elbow. Then I roll him over. Then I change rooms.
—ROAMING IN FORT WORTH

CHAPTER SEVEN

CPAP—The Best But Maybe Too Much

You now know enough about the collapse of your upper airway to go on *Jeopardy,* if the show had a category called soft tissue. It is time to learn about treatments and we'll review the full range: all the ones that come from doctors and all the ones you can send for that may or may not be junk mail.

Let's start at the top. The *only* treatment for snoring, whether apnea or just annoying, that *always* works is a machine called CPAP, which stands for continuous positive airway pressure. I can't imagine what continuous *negative* airway pressure would be—vacuuming your throat perhaps—but I'll go along with the name of this device because, as one doctor told me, "It's the gold of snoring treatments."

The CPAP machine is a small portable generator that pumps air through the nose and into the upper airway to hold the tissues apart. With a pressure that can be adjusted, the blower sends a steady stream of air through a flexible hose and into a soft plastic mask that covers your nose and is held by head straps. Your doctor will determine how much pressure is needed to keep your airway tissues from collapsing.

CPAP keeps the passage open, but it doesn't *eliminate* the obstructions that cause snoring, so it must be used all night, every night. Although more effective than any other treatment, it does have a possible problem: unless you don't mind going to sleep dressed as a scuba diver, you might find it claustrophobic to have a mask strapped to your head with an anchored hose. There is no point in replacing snoring with a panic attack, although some women might feel that a panic attack is a more acceptable sound.

Moreover, suppose you're a snorer who is not an annoying husband but an eager bachelor with company making her first visit to your bed? Will the fires of romance burn for her when she embraces Hosehead? Your lips will be clear of the mask; but to kiss them, she will have to be upside down to have a place for her nose below your chin. It may be the first new sexual position since the Kama Sutra.

My own problem with CPAP would be a less romantic one: I always have to get out of bed to relieve myself at least once a night. Either I would have to whip off the mask like a superhero becoming a civilian or I would have to drag the blower behind me, like a full-bladdered Frankenstein.

In spite of these considerations, CPAP is just about foolproof, unless your *nasal* passage is also blocked. If you have allergies or other nasal problems, these should be treated first. CPAP can cause drying in the nose, so you might want to use it in combination with a vaporizer or humidifier. Your bedroom then might sound like a runway at O'Hare and your partner might want to return to the sound of snoring.

The thought of O'Hare triggers the thought that the CPAP machine is extra baggage for you to carry and for an airline to lose.

"The airline has lost my continuous positive airway pressure," you will say to the clerk.

"Of course," she'll reply. "That operates only during the flight."

If you find the CPAP mask uncomfortable, talk to your doctor about adjusting it. If you find the cost of CPAP uncomfortable—about $2,000—talk to your insurance company about help. The machine can be leased; but buying one makes more sense than leasing one for thirty-five years. I presume you want to stop snoring for more than three weeks because I presume you want to keep the same wife.

To get CPAP, you *must* have a doctor's prescription that follows a sleep study. Some snorers with apnea who need CPAP might find the device so oppressive that they would rather consider kicking the habit of sleeping. For people who have never been fond of an eighty-mile-an-hour wind blowing into their noses all night, people who don't want to feel like basketballs being inflated, there is a version of CPAP called Biphasic Nasal CPAP or BIPAP, which has a gentler pressure; and there is a still gentler one called RAMP. Your doctor will have to decide if your snoring can be stopped by a breeze instead of a gale.

BIPAP is more comfortable because it is two pressures rather than one. There is a drop in pressure when the sleeper exhales, a cycling that gives him a chance to start breathing in sync with the machine. And the third version, RAMP, begins at a low level of pressure and then increases to let the snorer fall asleep without a wind in his face.

CPAP doesn't cure the causes of snoring, but just a month of it raises the oxygen saturation of the blood. This dramatic result, combined with the guaranteed elimination of snoring, makes CPAP the gold standard of treatments. Some doctors, however, feel that the gold is tarnished because CPAP can be waiting to exhale.

"BIPAP and RAMP are no problem," says Dr. Dennis R. Bailey, a New Jersey dentist who treats snoring. "But *CPAP* . . . Well, just try to exhale against an air flow of sixty miles an hour; it can be work. Moreover, after about a month of it, many people feel better, feel rested, and go off it; long-term use of CPAP is very rare. And just one day off it can set you *back* that whole month. And there's one more thing. The biggest problem in snoring isn't for the snorer but the bed partner. With CPAP, instead of the snoring, the partner has to listen to a motor running all night."

However, the motor is white sound, a steady hum that seems preferable to the unnerving syncopation of snoring.

"Would you rather spend the night listening to a motor or to me?" I asked Judy.

"A motor would be Mozart compared to you," she replied. "And if I couldn't get a motor, a tape of the Battle of Midway would be fine."

In response to Dr. Bailey, Dr. Gabriele M. Barthlen, former director of the Sleep Study Clinic of New York's Mount Sinai Hospital, says, "Yes, CPAP is cumbersome and it's another sound and many people don't stick with it, but it's the only nonsurgical treatment that always works for apnea. And it should be *used* only for apnea. For average snoring, it's overkill, like shooting flies with a gun. Average snoring can be *prevented* by behavior modification: weight loss, no alcohol at night, no smoking at night, getting rid of nasal congestion, and not sleeping on your back."

And so, before you turn to the heavy weather of CPAP, make sure your snoring *requires* it and not merely the change of habits that Dr. Barthlen describes. For apnea, CPAP is ideal. For lesser snoring, it is unnecessarily and grandiosely blowing your nose.

Sam's snore is so deep and loud that the whole bed vibrates. It's like a vibrating bed in a cheap motel.

—In Motion in Albany

CHAPTER EIGHT

From the Mail And the Mall. Does Anything Work?

Is there anything that works as well against snoring as blowing your nose in reverse? Before I answer that question by considering the next big medical device, the dental appliance or jaw positioner, let's look at some things you can get from a drugstore, a catalog, or a garage sale. Every year in America, doctors, dentists, and medical supply houses sell $200 million worth of anti-snoring gadgets and treatments.

"Competition is intense and growing wildly," says Timothy Carr, marketing director of Distar, Inc., which makes the TheraSnore jaw positioner, one of about thirty such devices that cost between $300 and $1,500.

We'll look at jaw positioners in the next chapter; I've always believed in postponing dental work. First, let's look at simpler things, some of which I have tested. The National Academy of Science seems not to be interested in my work, but Judy feels it's of cosmic importance. Of course, I didn't test these devices in precisely the way that the NAS might have wanted. I don't know the size of my airway or the degree of my snoring, for Judy has never made a tape of it.

"I'm not sure it belongs with the girls' graduations and dance recitals," she has said. "As unforgettable as it is, of course."

Moreover, my height and weight are no indication of how I snore. As Dr. Neil B. Kavey says, "You can have a big man with a little airway and a little man with a big airway."

In saying "a little man with a big airway," Dr. Kavey isn't talking about a short president of Delta, but about the need for a sleep study before you try such drastic and expensive cures as laser surgery, an irreversible procedure that will be explained in the pages to come.

At a cost of five dollars for a box of ten, a Breathe Right strip, which claims to "open the nasal passages to reduce airflow resistance," can be bought at a drugstore or by calling 1-800-858-NOSE. Made in three sizes, Junior/Small, Small/Medium, and Medium/Large, the strip is a bandage that flares open the nostrils.

On the night I put one on, I not only enjoyed the macho look, as if I had been in a brawl, but I did seem to feel a little more air coming into my nose. Would that extra intake reduce or stop my snoring?

The answer came from Judy at dawn.

"You sounded about the same," she said. "Maybe a bandage isn't enough for you. Maybe you need a tourniquet."

"Yes, Dr. Kavey said that the strip may not make any difference. There's no literature on it."

However, the report of my friend, Dennis, a bachelor in Los Angeles, may not be literature, but it's a pertinent paragraph.

"The Breathe Right strip works for me," he said. "Every time a lady comes to spend the night, I use one."

"Does the strip totally stop your snoring?"

"Definitely softens it. You just can't let it bother you that you're looking silly."

Silly? A bandage on the nose is a conservative fashion statement when compared to the ball-on-the-back, which is worn to keep the snorer from sleeping on his back. Originally called Dr. Jonah's Snore Begone, this device is as old as America: at the time of the Revolution, the wife of a snorer sometimes sewed a small cannonball to the back of his nightshirt to discourage him from taking the position most conducive to snoring.

Variations on this device have been appearing since the days when George Washington was our First Snorer. In 1900, Leonidas Wilson patented a leather harness that strapped a multipronged object between the snorer's shoulder blades, a device that should have been called The Torquemada. Of the more than 300 anti-snoring inventions registered in the U.S. Patent Office, most of them are based on this principle, although one of the others could be called The Torquemada, Two: an electronic device that delivers a shock to the sleeper when he starts to snore. Does it stop your snoring or just make you less crazy than you were at bedtime?

There is also no literature on the cannonball-on-the-back, but there must have been a considerable amount of unmeasured profanity. A man forced to wear munitions to bed was probably so annoyed that he wished the cannonball were en route to his wife.

From Nicolet Biomedical, Inc., of Palatine, Illinois, at a cost of $25, I bought a dark blue T-shirt with three pockets in the back for tennis balls and WE'RE ON YOUR SIDE on the front. It was going to sleep in a uniform.

The goal of the ball-bearing nightshirt is the timeless one:

snorer rotation. From the moment that the first Pleistocene woman used her semi-simian elbow to nudge her sleeping mate and say, "If you don't stop that godawful noise, I'm gonna throw you back into the slime," the goal has been to move the snorer into a silent position. My testing this shirt, however, would have been an exercise in stupidity. Because I never sleep on my back but do all my snoring in the ideal anti-snoring position, three Dunlops on my spine would have made sense only if I were preparing to serve. And if I reversed the shirt and put the balls beneath me while lying on my stomach, then I would be awake all night, wondering why I was trying to sleep on tennis balls.

And so I dropped the tennis balls and moved on to a position-changer that was high tech: I would test the effect on my snoring of my being nudged electronically by the Sharper Image's Ultra Snore Control, a thirteen-dollar "silent" wrist alarm. When you snore with this device on your wrist, the sound triggers not a noise but a vibration on your skin that interrupts your snoring and makes you move to a new position. But how long will you hold this new position when your natural one keeps beckoning to you?

For me, this silent alarm would have been as pointless as the tennis balls. Would I have wanted it to turn me on my *back*, where world-class snoring was done? Nevertheless, one night I did try the Ultra Snore Control; and because I'm a light sleeper, its vibrations awakened me about two A.M., a signal to change my position. The problem was, of course, that I couldn't sleep in any other position. Snoring on my stomach was not just the only comfortable position for me: it was a feat I had polished through the years. I took pride in being able to snore in the best non-snoring position.

Just before five A.M., the vibrations awoke me again. This time, I did change my position: from the bed to the kitchen, where I had an early breakfast, for I knew there would be no more sleep. And here is a way that Ultra Snore Control *can* work: it wakes you up, makes you angry, and one cause of snoring—being asleep—is gone.

Another mail-order product with the potential to eliminate going to sleep as a cause of snoring is the Comfort Zone Silent Sleeper for nine dollars from Sears, a pillow guaranteed to "let you and your sleeping partner sleep in uninterrupted silence." Made of foam, it is meant to give neck support when you lie on your back, thus elevating your neck.

In spite of my being unable to sleep on my back with *any* pillow, I did try lying on a Comfort Zone Silent Sleeper and discovered that the neck was not meant to be elevated unless accompanied by the head. I felt as though somebody was about to wash my hair.

In addition to the tennis balls, the alarm, and the sleep-defying pillow, there are two other kinds of mail-order treatments: nasal sprays and nasal inserts. You would, however, do just as well to treat your snoring with prayer.

The sprays are such items as Y-Snore, which calls itself "a simple, natural, painless solution." A solution it is: it is definitely not a solid; but Dr. Gabriele M. Barthlen, the noted sleep disorders specialist, says it does nothing for snoring.

"An ancient Chinese homeopathic treatment," says the text, "Y-Snore is made from 100% all-natural herbs and it has no side effects."

It has no main effects, either. After inventing gunpowder, the Chinese should have quit when they were ahead. Gunpowder, not these drops, would clear the nose, though the drops are cheaper: $13 for a three-week supply. The drops, however, do have one thing in common with gunpowder: they burn.

"Nonprescription nasal drops, like the salines, don't stop snoring," says Dr. Barthlen. "A bedtime nasal decongestant can be of some help, but it has to be a *prescription* one, like a steroid. Afrin spray is the only good commercial one, but you can't use it for more than three or four consecutive nights or it loses its potency *and* causes addiction."

Because no nation on earth fleeces consumers as creatively as America, our drugstores and catalogs sell not only sprays that are good just for moistening plants, but also clips and coils that are inserted into the nostrils to widen them and thus stop snoring. There is Breathe Fit, a horseshoe-shaped device for $13; Breathe EZ, a U-shaped insert for $20; and Nozovent, a $15 device that also spreads the nostrils from the inside.

And there is Snore Stop 2000, a U-shaped rubber ring from the Walter Drake catalog. The catalog doesn't give the meaning of 2000. Perhaps it's the date when the ring might start working.

"*All* those nasal inserts are worthless," says Dr. Barthlen. "In fact, they move you *backward*. Not only don't they stop snoring, they probably make it worse because they partially block the flow of air. Anything that takes up space in the nose is a bad idea."

Another sleep disorders specialist makes another basic point.

"Most anti-snoring devices haven't undergone clinical testing," says Dr. Michael Thorpy, director of the Sleep-Wake Disorder Center at New York's Montefiore Hospital.

And so, snoring in America has produced more than one racket. ABC News says that the nation now has twenty-one million social snorers—give or take twenty million, for surveys of bedroom noises are not science's most reliable figures. Sales figures, however, are certifiably celestial.

"Anti-snoring products are booming," says a spokesman for Eckerd, the drugstore chain that sells Breathe Right, Y-

Snore, Snor Ban (a plastic jaw retainer), and also Snore No More herbal tablets—sixty of them for $50.

The spokesman speaks truth: There are now hundreds of products: drops, pills, inserts, herbs, bandages, balls, and a second pillow, the Snore-No-More, which claims to "position the head and neck to keep the airway open and prevent the tongue from falling back." The Snore-No-More clearly has the potential to fight sleep as effectively as the Comfort Zone Silent Sleeper.

When the Good Housekeeping Institute tested Breathe Right strips, Breathe EZ clips, Snore No More tablets, Snore No More drops, and the Snore-No-More pillow (one yearns for a product called Rhyme No More) on forty-three snorers for a month, the results were not encouraging. Less than 35 percent of the sleepmates of these snorers noticed a significant improvement from the use of the clips, the drops, and the pillow. About half the sleepmates said the tablets had helped. Only the strips scored well: 73 percent.

This test, of course, was semi-science. Would anything continue to work for *more* than a month? Remember what Dr. Barthlen said about Afrin nasal spray: it will give you no more than one quiet weekend. And remember her feeling about *all* of the drugstore stuff: Snore Not For.

In the Institute test, some of the snorers said that the pillow made no difference if you slept on your stomach or your side; one man said that when he removed the Breathe Right strip, he felt as though he were ripping off his nose; and another man said that the clips kept falling out of his nose and he couldn't find them in the morning.

There was no reason to look.

Because Breathe Right strips had scored highest, I ignored the doubts of the doctors and tried one a second time to see if the answer for me *was* merely to enlarge my nasal passages. At bedtime one night, I took another strip from a box of ten and pasted it halfway down my nose. And then, with tape on my head and hope in my heart, I turned to the woman beside me in bed, who happened to be Judy, and said, "Honey, if it's no trouble, would you try to listen to me all night?"

Her reply had religious feeling: "Why should this night be different from all other nights?"

When I awoke in the morning, Judy was trying to sneak in a nap; but I knew she would want me to wake her so that she could tell me my score.

"Well?" I said, giving her a loving shake. "Am I cured?"

With a moan, she pulled the blanket over her head.

"No use trying to hide," I said. "I know you're in there."

"This must've been something that Dante wrote about," she said.

"Just tell me how I *did*. Will you finally be able to get more sleep than Lady Macbeth?"

"Well," she said, surfacing, "you *were* softer until about three o'clock. After that, it seemed just about the same. You know what I think I'll do?"

"Don't leave me! We have too many things besides the snoring."

"I think I'll buy one of those electronic devices that makes the sound of the surf or a mortar attack and enjoy that instead."

"No, let's try the bandage *again*. If it worked till three, then maybe I just need *two* strips to make it through the whole night. Hmmm . . . I wonder if they should be on *top* of each other or side-by-side."

"Have you thought about the mummy look?"

And so, the following bedtime, I bandaged again and bade Judy a "Goodnight" that had a certain hollow ring.

In the morning, I pounced on the poor darling again.

"And *last* night?" I said.

"You were softer till about three," she said. "Then it was the same old you: an earful."

Breathe Right strips were the answer for me only if I decided that four hours of sleep would be enough or if Judy would be willing to find new accommodations at three A.M.

At about the same time as the Good Housekeeping tests, the Center for Research in Sleep Disorders in Cincinnati used polysomnographs to determine the effects of external nasal dilation on nine mild snorers. After two nights of study, both snoring severity and frequency improved because of increased nasal air flow from wearing Breathe Right strips over the bridges of their noses.

An encouraging little test, but keep it in perspective: just nine mild snorers for two nights in Cincinnati. All the bandages at Johnson & Johnson wouldn't help *one* man with apnea or even one who snored severely.

Neither the Good Housekeeping Institute nor the center in Cincinnati tested the two snore fighters that have become as popular as Breathe Right strips: jaw positioners and tongue retainers. Most varieties of these devices force the jaw forward in small increments according to need; but if you buy one from a drugstore, it's your brain that needs an increment.

"Don't ever consider over-the-counter oral appliances," says Robert Rogers, president of Pittsburgh's Dental Sleep Disorder Society. "Things like SnorBan and TheraSnore. They can give you joint pain, loose teeth, and muscle spasms."

Partly in agreement with Dr. Rogers is R. Michael Alvarez, a California dentist who feels that locking the jaw into position is a mistake, a feeling that is behind my own belief in tetanus shots.

"It's better to get right to the real culprit—the tongue," he says.

The real culprit, however, may be Alvarez himself, whose Snor-X device is a sheath that holds the tongue in place with suction and makes Dr. Barthlen shake her own head. Nevertheless, Alvarez is probably right when he says that Snor-X is better than a rival tongue retainer called Tongue Master, which forces the tongue to protrude between the teeth like a guillotine.

If you bite off your tongue during the night, you have certainly found a cure for snoring; but if you would rather not try that, then go to a dentist who specializes in sleep disorders, for any oral appliance *must* be fitted by him or her to your particular facial configuration. Would you get orthodontia at Kmart?

He woke me up just kicking me. I hit him with my pillow and took off for another room.

—HIT AND RUN IN PITTSBURGH

CHAPTER NINE

A Dental Answer— Without the Gale

Because dental appliances come in different styles and work in different ways, you shouldn't get one from a catalog or a garage sale but from a dentist or orthodontist who has been trained in the use of this device. When a dental appliance is being fitted, adjustments have to be made, including your adjustment to sleeping with something that will discourage the kissing of your newly silent face during the night. If someone put her tongue in your mouth when you were wearing a dental appliance, she might get only part of it back. And you will be dangerous every night, for this device, like CPAP, does not cure the physiological conditions that cause snoring. Most of the time, however, it does stop the noise.

Dental appliance therapy was in use as far back as the early 1900s, but only recently has it reached a level of excellence. Of the more than thirty different dental appliances now in use, let's forget twenty-eight and consider the two best: the mandibular advancement device, which brings the lower jaw forward, and the tongue retainer, which holds the tongue still in a forward position. Moreover, certain models of these appliances perform both of these functions at the same time and lift a drooping soft palate as well. None of them cleans your teeth.

The tongue retainer is a piece of soft plastic with a bulb that attaches to the tongue by suction and pulls it forward so it can't fall back into the airway. The problem with this device, however, is that snorers seem to be able to wear it for only three or four hours a night; and then, either the device loses its suction or they lose their patience. How long can anyone stick out his tongue?

Both more popular and more effective is the mandibular advancement device, which fits over the teeth and pulls the jaw forward, thus pulling forward the tongue, the tissues, and anything else lying around that could collapse while you're asleep on your back. You might look like early Jerry Lewis, but you'll look that way in the dark and your airway will be blessedly open.

To wear the jaw advancer, you must have enough healthy teeth to support it. If you don't have those teeth, then you'll have to use the tongue retainer, for which the only requirement is a healthy tongue.

"The oral appliance should be considered the first line of treatment before an invasive procedure like surgery," says New Jersey dentist Dr. Dennis R. Bailey, who says the cost of such a device can range from $500 to $2,000. Other dentists do admit that there is some discomfort in sleeping with a foreign device in your mouth, but the discomfort is usually brief and minor. There also can be increased salivation and there is even the slight possibility of gagging. No, there is no possibility that you'll be needing the Heimlich maneuver by your partner.

One woman I know is married to a man who has refused to believe that he snores. In desperation one night, she made a tape recording of his snoring. His response was heartfelt: he accused her of sleeping with another man. This husband's denial of snoring was so strong that it anesthetized his brain: he became the first man to ever think that a wife would give evidence of cheating to her own husband.

Moreover, the denial of snoring women is just as strong. A woman will admit to everything from shoplifting to extraterrestrial sex; but *snoring* . . .

"It's *unfeminine*," one of them told me, a woman who has given her husband an ultimatum about snoring: Stop accusing her of it.

"I guess I was wrong," he told me. "It must be locusts."

And so, this is the depth of the problem of snoring that is being attacked by CPAP, dental devices, nasal clips, nasal sprays, nasal bandages, laser surgery, wrist alarms, and tennis balls. And the attack keeps growing more intense. For example, one woman to whom I lent my tennis ball shirt has been experimenting with other anti-snoring sports.

"Tennis balls are so annoying that they make me turn right over to my stomach," she said, "but whiffle golf balls don't work: you can sleep on them."

This is experimentation that the Nobel prize committee seems to ignore, a foolish oversight, for it is the only experimentation that combines science and peace.

Before you get an oral device from a dentist or orthodontist, you should be examined by an otolaryngologist to make sure you have a clear nasal airway because the device will block your mouth. Nasal polyps, allergies, and a deviated septum are all potential blockers, but the effect of a nose ring on snoring is unknown. Its effect on *me* is to make me wonder if evolution is headed back the other way.

If your nose is clear, then a dental device can help you, no matter what kind of snoring you do: social, hypopnea, or apnea. For people with apnea who can't tolerate CPAP and don't want surgery, a dental device is the answer. It must be a perfect fit or it will advance the jaw too much or too little; and if too much, it might cause dental misalignment.

Ah, dental misalignment. What memories such crookedness brings back to me and what feeling I have for anyone wearing a dental device. When I was a teenager and needed orthodontia, I had to sleep with a retainer, a plastic device that kept my teeth from relocating. I did not fervently want straight teeth. I fervently wanted to kill the orthodontist, preferably slowly by cementing his mouth shut.

Nevertheless, a dental device is a good alternative to CPAP. Less uncomfortable, it is effective up to 85 percent of the time for mild-to-moderate apnea—*if* the snorer can breathe through his nose.

"I breathe through my nose, I'm skinny, I sleep on my stomach, and I *still* snore," I told Dr. Bailey. "Should I join a circus or give myself to a medical school?"

"Oh, there are snorers who sleep on their stomachs," he said. "And skinny ones who breathe through their noses."

"So what should I *do*? I have a daughter in college, so I have about thirty-five dollars to treat my snoring. CPAP and your device are out—unless insurance will cover them."

"I'm afraid not. Unless it's apnea, snoring is considered a social problem and not a medical condition, so insurance companies won't pay for dental devices."

"And Dr. Barthlen says to forget about clips and sprays. What about that new Chinese herb?"

"It'll dry you up like a prune. People who take it wake up craving water."

"So what's the cure for me?"

"The only *cure* is surgery. Everything else is management, and excellent management is a dental device that repositions the jaw—like this one, The Silencer."

He held up two clear plastic molds, an upper and lower, that reminded me of ones my orthodontist had used to take impressions with wet cement that dripped down my throat. For a moment, I reminisced about gagging.

"That's the *best* one?" I said.

"Yes, this one advances the jaw just enough to open the airway. It has a soft inner surface, it's very adjustable, and it's kind to the temporomandibular joint."

"Good: I've always had a deep feeling for that joint. What's the cost?"

"Well, the lab fee is about five hundred dollars and the dentist's fee usually matches that, so you're approaching the cost of CPAP—but without the claustrophobia."

"But Dr. Barthlen says that CPAP would be overkill for me and maybe the dental device would be, too. You see, I don't have apnea, so—"

"How do you *know* that?"

"My internist says so."

"Have you had a sleep study?"

"Do you know one for thirty-five bucks? Anyway, my doctor never said I needed one."

"You know how long an internist spends studying snoring in medical school?"

"It's an elective, right?"

"One they never take. Has your internist ever routinely asked you about snoring during your physical? Of course not; they never do. Tell me, do you ever feel daytime sleepiness, headache, impotence, or depression?"

"Just from that question; you're scaring me."

"You may well be just a social snorer. But I do want you to know that this is the only medical problem that's discussed more in cartoons than examining rooms. Snoring is really America's closet malady."

* * *

And so, what was the answer for a skinny, tennis-playing, nondrinking, drug-free, stomach-sleeping snorer who didn't need CPAP, couldn't afford a dental device, and wasn't interested in the affordably worthless?

The silent alarm told me only that it wasn't time to get up.

The tennis balls told me only that Dunlop made a lousy mattress.

The nasal bandage told me only that I'd be looking cool while I snored.

Whatever the answer for me might be, it was time to explore laser surgery, perhaps a greater gift from France than the Statue of Liberty. How many marriages has the Statue of Liberty saved?

I taped him and then played it for friends.
  "What the hell is that?" one of them said.
  Someone else said that it might be an animal mating call.
                    —THINKING OF DARWIN IN DENVER

CHAPTER TEN

Two Answers For Apnea: The Knife and the Laser

All right, let's chase to the cut.

If the snoring is either social or mild-to-moderate apnea, the only *cure* for it is surgery that cuts away the uvula, soft palate, and tonsils. If, however, the blockage is a very thick tongue that is deep in the throat, then the surgery might end the snoring but not the apnea; and *silent* apnea can mean a permanently silent night, unless the snorer's wife doesn't happen to mind spending the night taking his pulse.

"In the worst apnea, it's the back of the tongue that falls against the back of the throat, and no one yet has found a way to shave that area," said Dr. Arlene H. Markowitz, a top New York otolaryngologist.

"I get conflicting figures for the success rate of this surgery," I told her. "Some doctors say it's as low as 35 percent; others say it's as high as 85. It feels like the stock market."

"The figure is probably closer to 55 percent," she said. "Snoring, as you know, can have multiple causes. If a surgeon picks his patients carefully and treats only those with the anatomical problems that the surgery addresses, he or she will have better statistics. If the surgery is done on *all* snorers, regardless of the cause, the statistics will be worse. Some people do best on CPAP, despite its limitations. Also, some studies follow patients only for the first few months. Some people do well initially, but after several years worsen again. A longer study usually has a lower success rate. And, unfortunately, aging continues despite the surgery, so the tissue sometimes sags again."

In other words, many surgeons wouldn't want a Mr. Pickwick, a Sancho Panza, or Huck Finn's friend Jim, all distinguished snorers of world letters; and they wouldn't have wanted a king of Tahiti such as Pomare I, Pomare II, or Pomare III, for *pomare* in Tahitian means "man who makes noise in his sleep." Even in paradise, the surf is not the only roar.

Scalpel surgery to remove throat obstructions is called uvulo-palatophrayngoplasty or UPPP. (Just pronouncing the word should be two credits at medical school.) Done at a hospital under general anesthesia, UPPP is cutting away the uvula, part of the soft palate, and sometimes the tonsils, too; the surgeon is sort of a Roto-Rooter man who is making the airway both wider and higher.

Often costing as much as $10,000, UPPP calls for a hospital stay of a day or two and a willingness to have a sore throat for several weeks. Other possible complications are bleeding, infection, tongue numbness, food or liquid flowing into the nasal cavity during swallowing, and a temporary or permanent voice change. For some people, snoring may be preferable to losing their vibrato and having their noses full of soup. Moreover, the loss of the soft palate means a nagging feeling of mucus in your throat for three or four months. UPPP patients, however, generally adjust to the postoperative discomforts, which also include throat swelling and the need to eat only soft foods for a few weeks.

Before having this surgery, you *must* have a sleep study to reveal the size of your airway, the thickness of your tissues, and the degree of your blockage. UPPP is not just a nip and a tuck. It gives new meaning to clearing your throat.

And so, if your snoring is either social or mild-to-moderate apnea, you can see the problem in finding a cure: either too little or too much. The mail-order remedies will probably relieve you only of cash and a scalpel may create a hole in your head that you don't need.

Fortunately, there is a new kind of surgery that's less severe: laser-assisted uvulopalatoplasty or LAUP, in which a laser vaporizes the flabby tissues to enlarge the airway. Done at a doctor's office under a local anesthetic injected directly into the throat, LAUP is usually done in steps of three-to-five sessions of about twenty minutes each, with a four-week recovery period between them. In each session, a small amount of tissue is vaporized with a pen-size device that makes the throat opening a little higher and a little wider: removed are part or all of the uvula and some of the soft palate, but not the tonsils or the base of the tongue.

Because laser surgery removes less tissue than a knife, the recovery period is shorter and the sore throat milder, although the complications are similar: a swollen throat, a temporary or permanent voice change, and food or liquid flowing into the nasal cavity when you swallow. If you don't want your dinner to be exploring your Eustachian tube, you'd better think twice about surgery. And LAUP, of course, is *not* enough tissue removal to cure severe apnea that is caused by a big, floppy tongue; and it is *not* for people whose snoring is caused by nasal congestion or by the irregularly shaped nasal passages of a deviated septum.

Developed in Paris in 1989 by Dr. Yves Victor Kamani, LAUP costs between $1,500 and $3,000 and is covered by insurance only if the patient's condition is apnea. This single exception is ironic because laser surgery may not cure apnea. It is excellent for a snorer whose problem is just a very large uvula and soft palate; but slicing the tongue is still a procedure that should be confined to making sandwiches.

An added warning comes from Dr. Jack Coleman of the Vanderbilt University Medical Center. In 1992, he became the first doctor to perform LAUP surgery in America.

"LAUP is a generally successful procedure," says Dr. Coleman, "but it does cause damage to the tissue and that tissue swells. So if a patient has apnea, the swelling could block the airway for a dangerous length of time and even cause death."

But let us not end this chapter on a downbeat note, for the outlook for snorers of every kind, as you have seen, is quite bright. Let's move on now to that brightness and review what *you* can do.

It sounds a little like—well, like the snort of a pig. But I don't want to live on a farm.

—DEVOUTLY URBAN IN NEW YORK

CHAPTER ELEVEN

Summing Up Your Options

And so, what have we learned?

If you are a social snorer and an otolaryngologist has studied you and found no obstructive sleep apnea, then the two best medical treatments, CPAP and surgery, might be overkill for you, as Dr. Gabriele M. Barthlen, the noted sleep disorders specialist, has said. If, however, you are a severe snorer *without* apnea, then LAUP is probably the right cure for you, although a dental device also might work.

As for all the drugstore treatments, remember what Dr. Barthlen has told us: every one of them, except perhaps a Breathe Right strip, would be a fling at futility. You can try the strips, of course—they are certainly cheap enough—but tests have revealed that about half the people who use them would do just as well with prayer.

For the social snorer, the answer seems to be a middle road between the surgeons and the snake-oil salesmen: get a dental device fitted just for you that will reposition your jaw when you sleep and end your snoring, a technique that

Dr. Dennis Bailey has described in Chapter Nine. As soon as my youngest daughter finishes college and my bank balance rises above $37.50, I may get such a device for myself.

If you're not a social snorer but a severe one and suspect that you may have apnea, you must go at once to an oto-laryngologist and have a sleep study.

"I cannot overemphasize the value of a sleep study," says Dr. Barthlen. "Only by having the snorer spend an entire night with a polysomnograph can we get a complete picture of the severity of the snoring and know whether apnea is present."

If it's apnea, you now know how dangerous that is. If you've forgotten, listen to Dr. David O. Goldfarb, chief of Otolaryngology at the Medical Center at Princeton, New Jersey: "The tendency of people with apnea to fall asleep without warning can be lethal. Research shows that the risk of being in an automobile accident is two to five times greater for sleep-apnea sufferers than for those who sleep normally."

As you now also know, LAUP has a *chance* of curing apnea, but is not a *guarantee*. The surgeon cannot predict with certainty; he or she can only give an educated guess after study of the apnea's precise degree. A dental device, however, is definitely not enough to unblock the airway of the apnea patient. Only CPAP *always* works.

No matter what kind of snoring you do, physical conditioning and certain changes in your presleep routine will lessen the snoring to some degree, according to every doctor who has contributed to this book. Dr. Riccardo A. Stoohs of the Stanford University Sleep Disorders Center spells it out.

"First," he says, "eat moderately and watch your weight. Research has shown a link between obesity and snoring because of extra fatty tissue at the throat of overweight men and women."

Every doctor has confirmed that nearly all people with apnea are overweight. In fact, a man can take the world's fastest physical just by looking inside his shirt collar, for Dr. William Demente, director of Sleep Disorder Study at Stanford, says, "Anyone with a neck of more than seventeen inches is at risk for sleep apnea."

And so, stop sending so much food past your uvula. Don't be a fathead: have a salad and make more room in your airway.

Also, try to confine your use of alcohol to cleaning wounds. Alcohol taken internally at bedtime reduces muscle tone during sleep even more than normal reduction. Some research says that the number of episodes of sleep apnea can actually double if you drink before going to bed.

Perhaps you feel that you need a drink before bedtime to relax. However, Dr. Michael J. Thorpy, director of New York's Sleep-Wake Disorders Center, says, "Alcohol may put you out, but it also can rob you of rest by disturbing your body's normal sleep patterns. And the same warning applies to sedatives and antihistamines at bedtime."

Sedatives and antihistamines relax the throat muscles; and when you go to sleep, every part of you should be relaxed *except* your throat. Of course, no one has ever figured out how to do that.

Furthermore, all the doctors say not to smoke, for tobacco irritates your upper airway and makes it congested. Instead of inhaling smoke at bedtime, you might try a nasal decongestant, but *only* one prescribed by your doctor, as Dr. Barthlen has said; the over-the-counter ones are no better than sniffing ginger ale. And remember that even a prescribed decongestant, while possibly reducing your snoring, won't come close to curing it.

Another thing you can do is change body positions during sleep: seek out non-snoring positions. A jab or shake from your beloved is excellent encouragement to do this. As you have learned, try not to sleep on your back. However, as you also have learned, more than half of back sleepers will snore just as nicely on their sides; and people with apnea will snore if they sleep standing up. Of course, going to sleep with the traditional ball-on-the-back *may* cure your snoring by keeping you up all night.

If you can sleep without a pillow, say the doctors, do so, for being perfectly flat helps to straighten your airway. A firm mattress also may help.

A firm body will help even more.

"Try to do regular workouts," says Dr. Michael Thorpy, "but *not* at night. Exercise revs up your whole system just when you want to be winding down. At bedtime, in fact, you might even try some deep breathing or relaxation exercise like yoga or tai chi."

With regular exercise, sensible eating, and little alcohol, try to get yourself in such good condition that you will live into a future where sleep studies will be done at home. Because many people don't feel comfortable spending a night at a sleep disorders center, there will soon be a portable polysomnograph to evaluate your snoring in your own bedroom. It will be an ideal gift for Father's Day.

Meanwhile, with whichever treatment you try, good luck. In some of the words of Dylan Thomas,

Do not go noisy into that good night.
Something in this book can keep your tissues tight.

AFTERWORD
All the Sleep Disorders Centers in America

ASDA MEMBER CENTERS AND LABORATORIES

ALABAMA

Brookwood Sleep Disorders
  Center
Brookwood Medical Center
2010 Brookwood Medical
  Center Drive
Birmingham, AL 35209

Sleep Disorders Center of
  Alabama, Inc.
790 Montclair Road, Suite 200
Birmingham, AL 35213

Sleep-Wake Disorders Center
University of Alabama at
  Birmingham
1713 6th Avenue South
CPM Building, Room 270
Birmingham, AL 35233-0018

Sleep-Wake Disorders Center
Flowers Hospital
4370 West Main Street
PO Box 6907
Dothan, AL 36302

Alabama North Regional Sleep
  Disorders Center
250 Chateau Drive, Suite 235
Huntsville, AL 35801

Huntsville Hospital Sleep
  Disorders Center
101 Sivley Road
Huntsville, AL 35801

Sleep Disorders Center
Mobile Infirmary Medical
  Center
PO Box 2144
Mobile, AL 36652

ALABAMA (Continued)

Southeast Regional Center for
Sleep/Wake Disorders
Springhill Memorial Hospital
3719 Dauphin Street
Mobile, AL 36608

USA Knollwood Sleep Disorders
Center
University of South Alabama
Knollwood Park Hospital
5600 Girby Road
Mobile, AL 36693-3398

Baptist Sleep Disorders Center
Baptist Medical Center
2105 East South Boulevard
Montgomery, AL 36116-2498

Tuscaloosa Clinic Sleep Lab
701 University Boulevard East
Tuscaloosa, AL 35401

ALASKA

Sleep Disorders Center
Providence Alaska Medical
Center
3200 Providence Drive
PO Box 196604
Anchorage, AK 99519-6604

ARIZONA

Samaritan Regional Sleep
Disorders Program
Desert Samaritan Medical Center
1400 South Dobson Road
Mesa, AZ 85202

Samaritan Regional Sleep
Disorders Program
Good Samaritan Regional
Medical Center
1111 East McDowell Road
Phoenix, AZ 85006

Sleep Disorders Center at
Scottsdale Memorial Hospital
Scottsdale Memorial Hospital-
North
10450 North 92nd Street
Scottsdale, AZ 85261-9930

Sleep Disorders Center
University of Arizona
1501 North Campbell Avenue
Tucson, AZ 85724

ARKANSAS

Sleep Disorders Center
Washington Regional Medical
Center
1125 North College Avenue
Fayetteville, AR 72703

Pediatric Sleep Disorders
Arkansas Children's Hospital
800 Marshall Street
Little Rock, AR 72202-3591

Sleep Disorders Center
Baptist Medical Center
9601 I-630, Exit 7
Little Rock, AR 72205-7299

CALIFORNIA

WestMed Sleep Disorders Center
1101 South Anaheim Boulevard
Anaheim, CA 92805

Mercy Sleep Laboratory
Mercy San Juan Hospital
6501 Coyle Avenue
Carmichael, CA 96508

Palomar Medical Center Sleep
    Disorders Lab
Palomar Medical Center
555 East Valley Parkway
Escondido, CA 92025

Sleep Disorders Institute
St. Jude Medical Center
100 East Valencia Mesa Drive
Suite 308
Fullerton, CA 92635

Glendale Adventist Medical
    Center Sleep Disorders
    Center
Glendale Adventist Medical
    Center
1509 Wilson Terrace
Glendale, CA 91206

Sleep Disorders Center
Scripps Clinic and Research
    Foundation
10666 North Torrey Pines Road
La Jolla, CA 92037

Sleep Disorders Center
Grossmont Hospital
PO Box 158
La Mesa, CA 91944-0158

Memorial Sleep Disorders Center
Long Beach Memorial Medical
    Center
2801 Atlantic Avenue
PO Box 1428
Long Beach, CA 90801-1428

Sleep Disorders Center
Cedars-Sinai Medical Center
8700 Beverly Boulevard
Los Angeles, CA 90048-1869

UCLA Sleep Disorders Center
710 Westwood Plaza
Los Angeles, CA 90095

Sleep Disorders Center
Hoag Memorial Hospital
    Presbyterian
301 Newport Boulevard
PO Box 6100
Newport Beach, CA 92658-6100

Sleep Evaluation Center
Northridge Hospital Medical
    Center
18300 Roscoe Boulevard
Northridge, CA 91328

California Center for Sleep
    Disorders
3012 Summit Street
5th Floor, South Building
Oakland, CA 94609

University of California, Irvine
Sleep Disorders Center
101 City Drive, Route 23
Orange, CA 92668

St. Joseph Hospital Sleep
    Disorders Center
1310 West Stewart Drive
Suite 403
Orange, CA 92668

Sleep Disorders Center
Huntington Memorial Hospital

CALIFORNIA (Continued)

100 West California Boulevard
PO Box 7013
Pasadena, CA 91109-7013

Sleep Disorders Center
Doctors Hospital - Pinole
2151 Appian Way
Pinole, CA 94564-2578

Pomona Valley Hospital Medical
Center
Sleep Disorders Center
1798 North Ganey Avenue
Pomona, CA 91767

The Center for Sleep Apnea
Redding Specialty Hospital
2801 Eureka Way
Redding, CA 96002

Sleep Disorders Center
Sequoia Hospital
170 Alameda de las Pulgas
Redwood City, CA 94062-2799

Sleep Disorders Center at
Riverside
Riverside Community Hospital
4445 Magnolia, E1
Riverside, CA 92501

Sutter Sleep Disorders Center
650 Howe Avenue
Suite 910
Sacramento, CA 95825

Mercy Sleep Disorders Center
Mercy HealthCare San Diego
4077 Fifth Avenue
San Diego, CA 92103-2180

San Diego Sleep Disorders
Center
1842 Third Avenue
San Diego, CA 92101

Sleep Disorders Center
California Pacific Medical
Center
2340 Clay Street, Suite 237
San Francisco, CA 94155

UCSF/Mt. Zion Sleep Disorders
Center
University of California, San
Francisco
1500 Divisadero Street
San Francisco, CA 94115

Sleep Disorders Center
San Jose Medical Center
675 East Santa Clara Street
San Jose, CA 95112

The Sleep Disorders Center of
Santa Barbara
2410 Fletcher Avenue
Suite 201
Santa Barbara, CA 93105

Sleep Disorders Clinic
Stanford University
401 Quarry Road
Stanford, CA 94305

Southern California Sleep Apnea
Center
Lombard Medical Group
2230 Lynn Road
Thousand Oaks, CA 91360

Torrance Memorial Medical
Center

Sleep Disorders Center
3330 West Lornita Boulevard
Torrance, CA 90505

Sleep Disorders Laboratory
Kaweah Delta District Hospital
400 West Mineral King Avenue
Visalia, CA 93291

West Hills Sleep Disorders
  Center
23101 Sherman Place
Suite 108
West Hills, CA 91307

Sleep Disorders Center
Woodland Memorial Hospital
1325 Cottonwood Street
Woodstand, CA 95695

COLORADO

National Jewish/University of
  Colorado Sleep Center
1400 Jackson Street, A200
Denver, CO 80206

CONNECTICUT

Danbury Hospital Sleep
  Disorders Center
Danbury Hospital
24 Hospital Avenue
Danbury, CT 06810

New Haven Sleep Disorders
  Center
100 York Street
University Towers
New Haven, CT 06511

Gaylord-Yale Sleep Disorders
  Laboratory
Gaylord Hospital
Gaylord Farms Road
Wallingford, CT 06492

DELAWARE

No Accredited Members

DISTRICT OF
COLUMBIA

Sleep Disorders Center
Georgetown University Hospital
3800 Reservoir Road, Northwest
Washington, DC 20007-2197

Sibley Memorial Hospital Sleep
  Disorders Center
5255 Loughboro Road Northwest
Washington, DC 20016

FLORIDA

Boca Raton Sleep Disorders
  Center
899 Meadows Road, Suite 101
Boca Raton, FL 33486

Sleep Disorder Laboratory
Broward General Medical Center
1600 South Andrews Avenue
Fort Lauderdale, FL 33316

Mayo Sleep Disorders Center
Mayo Clinic Jacksonville
4500 San Pablo Road
Jacksonville, FL 32224

FLORIDA (Continued)

Center for Sleep Disordered
  Breathing
PO Box 2982
Jacksonville, FL 32203

Watson Clinic Sleep Disorders
  Center
The Watson Clinic
1600 Lakeland Hills Boulevard
PO Box 95000
Lakeland, FL 33804-5000

Atlantic Sleep Disorders Center
1401 South Apollo Boulevard
Melbourne, FL 32901

Sleep Disorders Center
Mt. Sinai Medical Center
4300 Alton Road
Miami Beach, FL 33140

Sleep Disorders Center
Miami Children's Hospital
6125 Southwest 31st Street
Miami, FL 33155

University of Miami School of
  Medicine, JMH and VA
  Medical Center Sleep
  Disorders Center
Department of Neurology (D4-5)
PO Box 016960
Miami, FL 33101

Florida Hospital Sleep Disorders
  Center
601 East Rollins Avenue
Orlando, FL 32803

Health First Sleep Disorders
  Center
Palm Bay Community Hospital
1425 Malabar Road Northeast
Suite 255
Palm Bay, FL 32907

Sleep Disorders Center
Sarasota Memorial Hospital
1700 South Tamiami Trail
Sarasota, FL 34239

St. Petersburg Sleep Disorders
  Center
2525 Pasadena Avenue South,
  Suite S
St. Petersburg, FL 33707

Laboratory for Sleep Related
  Breathing Disorders
University Community Hospital
3100 East Fletcher Avenue
Tampa, FL 33613

GEORGIA

Sleep Disorders Center of
  Georgia
5505 Peachtree Dunwoody Road
Suite 370
Atlanta, GA 30342

Sleep Disorders Center
Northside Hospital
1000 Johnson Ferry Road
Atlanta, GA 30342

Atlanta Center for Sleep Disorders
303 Parkway
Box 44
Atlanta, GA 30312

Sleep Disorders Center
Promina Kenneratone Hospital
677 Church Street
Marietta, GA 30060

Department of Sleep Disorders
    Medicine
Candler Hospital
5353 Reynolds Street
Savannah, GA 31405

Sleep Disorders Center
Memorial Medical Center, Inc.
4700 Waters Avenue
Savannah, GA 31403

Savannah Sleep Disorders Center
Saint Joseph's Hospital
#6 St. Joseph's Professional
    Plaza
11706 Mercy Boulevard
Savannah, GA 31419

HAWAII

Pulmonary Sleep Disorders
    Center
Kuakini Medical Center
347 North Kuakini Street
Honolulu, HI 96817

Sleep Disorders Center of the
    Pacific
Straub Clinic & Hospital
888 South King Street
Honolulu, HI 96813

IDAHO

No Accredited Members

ILLINOIS

Neurological Testing Center's
    Sleep Disorders Center
Northwestern Memorial Hospital
303 East Superior, Passavant
    1044
Chicago, IL 60611

Sleep Disorder Service and
    Research Center
Rush-Presbyterian-St. Luke's
1563 West Congress Parkway
Chicago, IL 60612

Sleep Disorders Center
The University of Chicago
    Hospitals
5841 South Maryland
MC2091
Chicago, IL 60637

Sleep Disorders Center
Evanston Hospital
2650 Ridge Avenue
Evanston, IL 60201

C. Duane Morgan Sleep
    Disorders Center
Methodist Medical Center of
    Illinois
221 Northeast Glen Oak Avenue
Peoria, IL 61636

SIU School of
    Medicine/Memorial Medical
    Center Sleep Disorders
    Center
Memorial Medical Center
800 North Rutledge
Springfield, IL 62781

ILLINOIS (Continued)

Carle Regional Sleep Disorders
  Center
Carle Foundation Hospital
611 West Park Street
Urbana, IL 61601-2595

INDIANA

St. Mary's Sleep Disorders
  Center
St. Mary's Medical Center
3700 Washington Avenue
Evansville, IN 47750

St. Joseph Sleep Disorders
  Center
St. Joseph Medical Center
700 Broadway
Fort Wayne, IN 46802

Sleep/Wake Disorders Center
Community Hospitals of
  Indianapolis
1500 North Ritter Avenue
Indianapolis, IN 46219

Sleep/Wake Disorders Center
Winona Memorial Hospital
3232 North Meridian Street
Indianapolis, IN 46208

Sleep Alertness Center
Lafayette Home Hospital
2400 South Street
Lafayette, IN 47904

Sleep Disorders Center
Good Samaritan Hospital
520 South 7th Street
Vincennes, IN 47591

IOWA

Sleep Disorders Center
Genesis Medical Center
1401 West Central Park
Davenport, IA 52804

Sleep Disorders Center
The Department of Neurology
The University of Iowa Hospitals
  and Clinics
Iowa City, IA 52242

KANSAS

Sleep Disorders Center
St. Francis Hospital and Medical
  Center
1700 Southwest 7th Street
Topeka, KS 66606-1690

Sleep Disorders Center
Wesley Medical Center
550 North Hillside
Wichita, KS 67214-4976

KENTUCKY

Sleep Lab
The Medical Center at Bowling
  Green
250 Park Street
PO Box 90010
Bowling Green, KY 42101-9010

Sleep Diagnostics Lab
Greenview Regional Medical
  Center
1801 Ashley Circle
Bowling Green, KY 42101

The Sleep Disorder Center of St.
Luke Hospital
St. Luke Hospital, Inc.
85 North Grand Avenue
Fort Thomas, KY 41075

Sleep Apnea Center
Columbia Hospital of Lexington
310 South Limestone
Lexington, KY 40508

Sleep Disorders Center
St. Joseph's Hospital
One St. Joseph Drive
Lexington, KY 40504

Sleep Disorders Center
Audubon Regional Medical
Center
One Audubon Plaza Drive
Louisville, KY 40217

Sleep Disorders Center
University of Louisville Hospital
530 South Jackson Street
Louisville, KY 40202

Regional Medical Center Lab for
Sleep-Related Breathing
Disorders
900 Hospital Drive
Madisonville, KY 42431

LOUISIANA

Mercy & Baptist Sleep Disorders
Center
2700 Napoleon Avenue
New Orleans, LA 70115

Tulane Sleep Disorders Center
1415 Tulane Avenue
New Orleans, LA 70112

LSU Sleep Disorders Center
Louisiana State University
Medical Center
PO Box 33932
Shreveport, LA 71130-3932

The Neurology and Sleep Clinic
2205 East 70th Street
Shreveport, LA 71105

MAINE

Maine Sleep Apnea Institute
Maine Medical Center
22 Bramhall Street
Portland, ME 04102

MARYLAND

The Johns Hopkins Sleep
Disorders Center
Asthma and Allergy Building,
Room 4850
Johns Hopkins Bayview Medical
Center
5501 Hopkins Bayview Circle
Baltimore, MD 21224

Maryland Sleep Disorders
Center, Inc.
Ruxton Towers, Suite 211
8415 Bellona Lane
Baltimore, MD 21204

Shady Grove Sleep Disorders
Center

MARYLAND (Continued)

14915 Broschart Road
Suite 102
Rockville, MD 20850

MASSACHUSETTS

Sleep Disorders Center
Beth Israel Hospital
330 Brookline Avenue KS430
Boston, MA 02215

Sleep Disorders Center
Lahey-Hitchcock Clinic
41 Mall Road
Burlington, MA 01805

Sleep Disorders Institute of
　　Central New England
St. Vincent Hospital
25 Winthrop Street
Worcester, MA 01604

MICHIGAN

Sleep/Wake Disorders
　　Laboratory (127B)
VA Medical Center
4646 John R.
Allen Park, MI 48202

Sleep Disorders Center
St. Joseph Mercy Hospital
PO Box 995
Ann Arbor, MI 48106

Sleep Disorders Center
University of Michigan Hospitals

1500 East Medical Center Drive
Med. Inn C433, Box 0842
Ann Arbor, MI 48109-0115

Sleep Disorders Clinic
Bay Medical Center
1900 Columbus Avenue
Bay City, MI 48708

Sleep Disorders Center
Henry Ford Hospital
2921 West Grand Boulevard
Detroit, MI 48202

Sleep Disorders Center
Butterworth Hospital
100 Michigan Street Northeast
Grand Rapids, MI 49503

Sleep Disorders Center
W.A. Foote Memorial Hospital,
　　Inc.
205 North East Avenue
Jackson, MI 49201

Borgess Sleep Disorders Center
Borgess Medical Center
1521 Gull Road
Kalamazoo, MI 49001

Michigan Capital Healthcare
　　Sleep/Wake Center
2025 South Washington Avenue
Suite 300
Lansing, MI 48910-0817

Sparrow Sleep Center
Sparrow Hospital
1215 East Michigan Avenue
PO Box 30480
Lansing, MI 48909-7980

Sleep Disorders Center
Oakwood Downriver Medical
    Center
25750 West Outer Drive
Lincoln Park, MI 48146-1599

Sleep & Respiratory Associates
    of Michigan
28200 Franklin Road
Southfield, MI 48034

Munson Sleep Disorders Center
Munson Medical Center
1105 6th Street
MPB Suite 307
Traverse City, MI 49684-2386

Sleep Disorders Institute
44199 Dequindre, Suite 311
Troy, MI 48096

MINNESOTA

Duluth Regional Sleep Disorders
    Center
St. Mary's Medical Center
407 East Third Street
Duluth, MN 55805

Sleep Disorders Center
Abbott Northwestern Hospital
800 East 28th Street at Chicago
    Avenue
Minneapolis, MN 55407

Minnesota Regional Sleep
    Disorders Center #8678
Hennepin County Medical Center
701 Park Avenue South
Minneapolis, MN 55415

Mayo Sleep Disorders Center
Mayo Clinic
200 First Street Southwest
Rochester, MN 55905

Sleep Disorders Center
Methodist Hospital
6500 Excelsior Boulevard
St. Louis Park, MN 55426

St. Joseph's Sleep Diagnostic
    Center
St. Joseph's Hospital
69 West Exchange Street
St. Paul, MN 55102

MISSISSIPPI

Sleep Disorders Center
Memorial Hospital at Gulfport
PO Box 1810
Gulfport, MS 39501

Sleep Disorders Center
Forrest General Hospital
PO Box 16389
6051 Highway 49
Hattiesburg, MS 39404

Sleep Disorders Center
University of Mississippi
    Medical Center
2500 North State Street
Jackson, MS 39216-4505

MISSOURI

Sleep Medicine and Research
    Center
St. Luke's Hospital
232 South Woods Mill Road
Chesterfield, MO 63017

MISSOURI (continued)

University of Missouri Sleep
    Disorders Center
M-741 Neurology
University Hospital and Clinics
One Hospital Drive
Columbia, MO 65212

Sleep Disorders Center
Research Medical Center
2316 East Meyer Boulevard
Kansas City, MO 64132

Sleep Disorders Center
St. Luke's Hospital
4400 Wornall Road
Kansas City, MO 64111

Cost Regional Sleep Disorders
    Center
3600 South National Avenue
Suite LL 150
Springfield, MO 65807

Sleep Disorders & Research
    Center
Deaconess Medical Center
6150 Oakland Avenue
St. Louis, MO 63139

Sleep Disorders Center
St. Louis University Medical
    Center
1221 South Grand Boulevard
St. Louis, MO 63104

MONTANA

No Accredited Members

NEBRASKA

Great Plains Regional Sleep
    Physiology Center
Lincoln General Hospital
2300 South 16th Street
Lincoln, NE 68502

Sleep Disorders Center
Clarkson Hospital
4350 Dewey Avenue
Omaha, NE 68105-1018

Sleep Disorders Center
Methodist/Richard Young
    Hospital
2566 St. Mary's Avenue
Omaha, NE 68105

NEVADA

The Sleep Clinic of Nevada
1012 East Sahara Avenue
Las Vegas, NV 89104

Regional Center for Sleep
    Disorders
Sunrise Hospital and Medical
    Center
3186 South Maryland Parkway
Las Vegas, NV 89109

Washoe Sleep Disorders Center
    and Sleep Laboratory
Washoe Professional Building
    and Washoe Medical Center
75 Pringle Way, Suite 701
Reno, NV 89502

NEW HAMPSHIRE

Sleep-Wake Disorders Center
Hampstead Hospital
East Road
Hampstead, NH 03841

Sleep Disorders Center
Dartmouth-Hitchcock Medical
Center
One Medical Center Drive
Lebanon, NH 03756

NEW JERSEY

Institute for Sleep/Wake
Disorders
Hackensack University Medical
Center
385 Prospect Avenue
Hackensack, NJ 07601

Sleep Disorder Center of
Morristown Memorial
Hospital
95 Mount Kemble Avenue
2nd Floor, Thebaud Building
Morristown, NJ 07962

Comprehensive Sleep Disorders
Center
Robert Wood Johnson University
Hospital
UMDNJ—Robert Wood Johnson
Medical School
One Robert Wood Johnson Place
PO Box 2601
New Brunswick, NJ 08903-2601

Sleep Disorders Center
Newark Beth Israel Medical
Center
201 Lyons Avenue
Newark, NJ 07112

Mercer Medical Center Sleep
Disorders Center
Mercer Medical Center
446 Bellevue Avenue
PO Box 1658
Trenton, NJ 06607

NEW MEXICO

University Hospital Sleep
Disorders Center
University of New Mexico
Hospital
4775 Indian School Road
Northeast
Suite 307
Albuquerque, NM 87110

NEW YORK

Capital Region Sleep/Wake
Disorders Center
St. Peter's Hospital and Albany
Medical Center
25 Hackett Boulevard
Albany, NY 12208

Sleep-Wake Disorders Center
Montefiore Medical Center
111 East 210th Street
Bronx, NY 10467

NEW YORK (Continued)

St. Joseph's Hospital Sleep
    Disorders Center
St. Joseph's Hospital
555 East Market Street
Elmira, NY 14902

Sleep Disorders Center
Winthrop-University Hospital
222 Station Plaza North
Mineola, NY 11501

Sleep-Wake Disorders Center
Long Island Jewish Medical
    Center
270-05 76th Avenue
New Hyde Park, NY 11042

The Sleep Disorders Center
Columbia Presbyterian Medical
    Center
161 Fort Washington Avenue
New York, NY 10032

Sleep Disorders Institute
St. Luke's/Roosevelt Hospital
    Center
1090 Amsterdam Avenue
New York, NY 10025

Sleep Disorders Center of
    Rochester
2110 Clinton Avenue South
Rochester, NY 14618

Sleep Disorders Center
State University of New York at
    Stony Brook
University Hospital

MR 120 A
Stony Brook, NY 11794-7139

The Sleep Center
Community General Hosptial
Broad Road
Syracuse, NY 13215

The Sleep Laboratory
945 East Genesee Street
Suite 300
Syracuse, NY 13210

Sleep-Wake Disorders Center
New York Hospital-Cornell
    Medical Center
21 Bloomingdale Road
White Plains, NY 10505

NORTH CAROLINA

Sleep Medicine Center of
    Asheville
1091 Hendersonville Road
Asheville, NC 28803

Sleep Center
University Hospital
PO Box 560727
Charlotte, NC 28256

Sleep Disorders Center
The Moses H. Cone Memorial
    Hospital
1200 North Elm Street
Greensboro, NC 27401-1020

Sleep Disorders Center
North Carolina Baptist Hospital

Bowman Gray School of
   Medicine
Medical Center Boulevard
Winston-Salem, NC 27157

Summit Sleep Disorders Center
160 Charlois Boulevard
Winston-Salem, NC 27103

NORTH DAKOTA

Sleep Disorders Center
MeritCare Hospital
720 4th Street North
Fargo, ND 58122

OHIO

Sleep Disorders Center
Bethesda Oak Hospital
619 Oak Street
Cincinnati, OH 45206

The Tri-State Sleep Disorders
   Center
1275 East Kemper Road
Cincinnati, OH 45246

Sleep Disorders Center
The Cleveland Clinic Foundation
9500 Euclid Avenue, Desk S-83
Cleveland, OH 44195

Sleep Disorders Center
Rainbow Babies Children's
   Hospital
Case Western Reserve University
11100 Euclid Avenue
Cleveland, OH 44106

Sleep Disorders Center
The Ohio State University
   Medical Center
Rhodes Hall, S1039
410 West 10th Avenue
Columbus, OH 43210-1228

The Center for Sleep & Wake
   Disorders
Miami Valley Hospital
One Wyoming Street
Suite G-200
Dayton, OH 45409

Ohio Sleep Medicine and
   Neuroscience Institute
4975 Bradenton Avenue
Dublin, OH 43017

Sleep Disorders Center
Kettering Medical Center
3535 Southern Boulevard
Kettering, OH 45429-1295

Sleep Disorders Center
St. Vincent Medical Center
2213 Cherry Street
Toledo, OH 43608-2691

Northwest Ohio Sleep Disorders
   Center
The Toledo Hospital
Harris-McIntosh Tower, Second
   Floor
2142 North Cove Boulevard
Toledo, OH 43606

Sleep Disorders Center
Good Samaritan Medical Center
800 Forest Avenue
Zanesville, OH 43701

OKLAHOMA

Sleep Disorders Center of
   Oklahoma
Southwest Medical Center of
   Oklahoma
4401 South Western Avenue
Oklahoma City, OK 73109

OREGON

Sleep Disorders Center
Sacred Heart Medical Center
1255 Hilyard Street
PO Box 10905
Eugene, OR 97440

Sleep Disorders Center
Rogue Valley Medical Center
2825 East Barnett Road
Medford, OR 97504

Neurology, N-450
Legacy Good Samaritan Sleep
   Disorders Center
1015 Northwest 22nd Avenue
Portland, OR 97210

Sleep Disorders Laboratory
Providence Medical Center
4805 Northeast Glisan Street
Portland, OR 97213

Salem Hospital Sleep Disorders
   Center
Salem Hospital
665 Winter Street Southeast
Salem, OR 97309-5014

PENNSYLVANIA

Sleep Disorders Center
Abington Memorial Hospital
1200 Old York Road
2nd Floor Rorer Building
Abington, PA 19001

Lehigh Valley Hospital Sleep
   Disorders Center
Lehigh Valley Hospital
Cedar Crest and I-78
PO Box 689
Allentown, PA 18105-1556

Sleep Disorders Center
Lower Bucks Hospital
501 Bath Road
Bristol, PA 19007

Sleep Disorders Center of
   Lancaster
Lancaster General Hospital
555 North Duke Street
Lancaster, PA 17604-3555

Sleep Disorders Center
Medical College of Pennsylvania
   and Hahnemann
3200 Henry Avenue
Philadelphia, PA 19129

Penn Center for Sleep Disorders
Hospital of the University of
   Pennsylvania
3400 Spruce Street, 11 Gates
   West
Philadelphia, PA 19104

Sleep Disorders Center
Thomas Jefferson University
1025 Walnut Street
Suite 316
Philadelphia, PA 19107

Pulmonary Sleep Evaluation
   Center

University of Pittsburgh Medical
Center
Montefiore University Hospital
3459 Fifth Avenue, S639
Pittsburgh, PA 15213

Sleep and Chronobiology Center
Western Psychiatric Institute and
Clinic
3811 O'Hara Street
Pittsburgh, PA 15213-2593

Sleep Disorders Center
Community Medical Center
1822 Mulberry Street
Scranton, PA 18510

Sleep Disorders Center
Crozer-Chester Medical Center
One Medical Center Boulevard
Upland, PA 19013-3975

Sleep Disorders Center
The Lankenau Hospital
100 Lancaster Avenue
Wynnewood, PA 19096

RHODE ISLAND

Sleep Disorders Center
Rhode Island Hospital
593 Eddy Street, APC-301
Providence, RI 02903

SOUTH CAROLINA

Roper SleepWake Disorders
Center
Roper Hospital
315 Calhoun Street
Charleston, SC 29401-1125

Sleep Disorders Center of South
Carolina
Baptist Medical Center
Taylor at Marion Streets
Columbia, SC 29220

Sleep Disorders Center
Greenville Memorial Hospital
701 Grove Road
Greenville, SC 29605

Children's Sleep Disorders
Center
Self Memorial Hospital
1325 Spring Street
Greenwood, SC 29646

Sleep Disorders Center
Spartanburg Regional Medical
Center
101 East Wood Street
Spartanburg, SC 29303

SOUTH DAKOTA

The Sleep Center
Rapid City Regional Hospital
353 Fairmont Boulevard PO Box
6000
Rapid City, SD 57709

Sleep Disorders Center
Sioux Valley Hospital
1100 South Euclid
Sioux Falls, SD 57117-5039

TENNESSEE

Sleep Disorders Laboratory
Regional Hospital of Jackson
367 Hospital Boulevard
Jackson, TN 38303

TENNESSEE (Continued)

Sleep Disorders Center
Ft. Sanders Regional Medical
   Center
1901 West Clinch Avenue
Knoxville, TN 37916

Sleep Disorders Center
St. Mary's Medical Center
900 East Oak Hill Avenue
Knoxville, TN 37917-4556

BMH Sleep Disorders Center
Baptist Memorial Hospital
899 Madison Avenue
Memphis, TN 38146

Sleep Disorders Center
Methodist Hospital of Memphis
1265 Union Avenue
Memphis, TN 38104

Sleep Disorders Center
Centennial Medical Center
2300 Patterson Street
Nashville, TN 37203

Sleep Disorders Center
Saint Thomas Hospital
PO Box 360
Nashville, TN 37202

TEXAS

NWTH Sleep Disorders Center
Northwest Texas Hospital
PO Box 1110
Amarillo, TX 79175

Sleep Disorders Center for
   Children
Children's Medical Center of
   Dallas
1935 Motor Street
Dallas, TX 75235

Sleep Medicine Institute
Presbyterian Hospital of Dallas
8200 Walnut Hill Lane
Dallas, TX 75231

Sleep Disorders Center
Columbia Medical Center West
1801 North Oregon
El Paso, TX 79902

Sleep Disorders Center
Providence Memorial Hospital
2001 North Oregon
El Paso, TX 79902

All Saints Sleep Disorders
   Diagnostic & Treatment
   Center
All Saints Episcopal Hospital
1400 8th Avenue
Fort Worth, TX 76104

Sleep Disorders Center
Department of Psychiatry
Baylor College of Medicine and
   VA Medical Center
One Baylor Plaza
Houston, TX 77030

Sleep Disorders Center
Spring Branch Medical Center
8850 Long Point Road
Houston, TX 77055

Sleep Disorders Center
Scott and White Clinic
2401 South 31st Street
Temple, TX 76508

UTAH

Intermountain Sleep Disorders
    Center
LDS Hospital
325 8th Avenue
Salt Lake City, UT 84143

University Health Sciences
    Center
Sleep Disorders Center
50 North Medical Drive
Salt Lake City, UT 84132

VERMONT

No Accredited Members

VIRGINIA

Fairfax Sleep Disorders Center
3289 Woodburn Road
Suite 360
Annandale, VA 22003

Sleep Disorders Center for
    Adults and Children
Eastern Virginia Medical School
Sentara Norfolk General Hospital
600 Gresham Drive
Norfolk, VA 23507

Sleep Disorders Center
Medical College of Virginia
PO Box 980710—MCV
Richmond, VA 23298-0710

Sleep Disorders Center
Community Hospital of Roanoke
    Valley
PO Box 12946
Roanake, VA 24029

WASHINGTON

Sleep Disorders Center for
    Southwest Washington
St. Peter Hospital
413 North Lilly Road
Olympia, WA 98506

Richland Sleep Laboratory
800 Swift Boulevard
Suite 260
Richland, WA 99352

Providence Sleep Disorders
    Center
Jefferson Tower
Suite 203
1600 East Jefferson
Seattle, WA 98122

Seattle Sleep Disorders Center
Swedish Medical Center/Ballard
PO Box 70707
Seattle, WA 98107-1507

Sleep Disorders Center
Virginia Mason Medical Center
PO Box 1930 Mail Stop H10-
    SDC
925 Seneca Street
Seattle, WA 98111-1930

Sleep Disorders Center
Sacred Heart Doctors Building
105 West Eighth Avenue

WASHINGTON
(continued)

Suite 418
Spokane, WA 99204

St. Clare Sleep Related Breathing
    Disorders Clinic
St. Clare Hospital
11315 Bridgeport Way
    Southwest
Tacoma, WA 98499

WISCONSIN

Regional Sleep Disorders Center
Appleton Medical Center
1818 North Meade Street
Appleton, WI 54911

Luther/Midelfort Sleep Disorders
    Center
Luther Hospital Midelfort Clinic
1221 Whipple Street
PO Box 4105
Eau Claire, WI 54702-4105

St. Vincent Hospital Sleep
    Disorders Center
St. Vincent Hospital
PO Box 13508
Green Bay, WI 54307-3508

Wisconsin Sleep Disorders
    Center
Gundersen Clinic, Ltd.
1836 South Avenue
La Crosse, WI 54601

Comprehensive Sleep Disorders
    Center

B6/579 Clinical Science Center
University of Wisconsin
    Hospitals and Clinics
600 Highland Avenue
Madison, WI 53792

Marshfield Sleep Disorders
    Center
Marshfield Clinic
1000 North Oak Avenue
Marshfield, WI 54449

Milwaukee Regional Sleep
    Disorders Center
Columbia Hospital
2025 East Newport Avenue
Milwaukee, WI 53211

Sleep/Wake Disorders Center
St. Luke's Sleep Disorders
    Center
St. Luke's Medical Center
2900 West Oklahoma Avenue
Milwaukee, WI 53201-2901

St. Mary's Hospital
2320 North Lake Drive
PO Box 503
Milwaukee, WI 53201-4565

WEST VIRGINIA

Sleep Disorders Center
Charleston Area Medical Center
501 Morris Street—PO Box
    1393
Charleston, WV 25325

WYOMING

No Accredited Members

INDEX

EPILOGUE

Just a few days before this book went to press, the FDA approved a new treatment for snoring called somnoplasty, which uses low frequency radio waves to shrink excess uvula and palate tissue that blocks the airway. Performed under local anesthesia in an outpatient suite, somnoplasty takes about a half hour.

But does it work?

Dr. Yosef P. Krespi, editor of this book says, "There seem to be three effects from the somnoplasty treatment: The excess tissue is reduced, the uvula is moved further from the tongue, and the palate is stiffened. However, somnoplasty has no effect on obstructive sleep apnea *and* there are as yet no proven long term results in curing even habitual snoring with radio waves. From my experience in treating more than one thousand snoring patients with a laser, it appears that such limited reduction of the uvula and palate can still result in a high incidence of recurrence."

In other words, the jury is still out. And some of them may be snoring. *Is* somnoplasty a new cure? It is still too early to know. And so, while we wait for proof of the treatment's value, you would be wiser to use one of the already proven cures in this book.

And *now* we can wish you a silent night.

By the year 2000, 2 out of 3 Americans could be illiterate.

It's true.

Today, 75 million adults… about one American in three, can't read adequately. And by the year 2000, U.S. News & World Report envisions an America with a literacy rate of only 30%.

Before that America comes to be, you can stop it… by joining the fight against illiteracy today.

Call the Coalition for Literacy at toll-free **1-800-228-8813** and volunteer.

Volunteer Against Illiteracy. The only degree you need is a degree of caring.

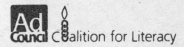

Ad Council Coalition for Literacy